Type 2 Diabetes Cookbook, Meals and Action Plan for Newly Diagnosed

The Ultimate Beginner's Diabetic Diet Cookbook, Meal and Action Plan – Reverse Diabetes with Proven, Easy and Healthy Recipes!

By Isabella Evelyn

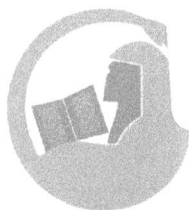

EFFINGO
Publishing

For more great books visit:

EffingoPublishing.com

Download another book for Free

We want to thank you for purchasing this book and offer you another book (just as long and valuable as this book), "Health & Fitness Mistakes You Don't Know You're Making," completely free.
Visit the link below to sign up and receive it:
www.effingopublishing.com/gift

In this book, we will break down the most common health & fitness mistakes, you are probably committing right now, and will reveal how you can easily get in the best shape of your life!

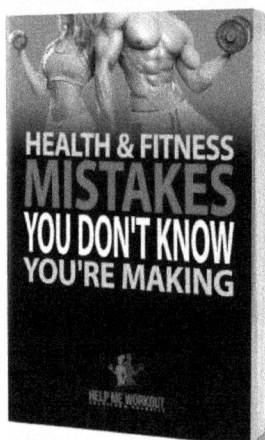

In addition to this valuable gift, you will also have an opportunity to get our new books for free, enter giveaways, and receive other valuable emails from us. Again, visit the link to sign up: **www.effingopublishing.com/gift**

TABLE OF CONTENTS

Introduction

It is undeniable that getting diagnosed with diabetes can be quite frightening, especially if you have no idea what to do after. Should you enroll in a specific exercise program? Should you drink a ton of medicine and supplements? Should you do this? Should you do that? There are are a lot of things to consider. However, the most overwhelming decision that you can make is what to eat.

Food is an essential part of our survival, and we love to eat. For a person with diabetes, this doesn't have to change. You do not have to sacrifice food for diabetes. All you need to do is change your prediabetes favorites into healthier options. The flavor is also not an issue because there are a lot of ways you can augment your meals to keep them flavorful yet healthier.

This is where the book, *Type 2 Diabetes Cookbook, Meals, and Action Plan for Newly Diagnosed*, comes in. This book will not only help you battle your way through diabetes with insights and helpful information but cook your way through as well. In this book, you will not only know ways to manage your meals and diet as a person with diabetes, but you will also have recipes and a sample one-month plan that you can use to help you go through your diabetes journey.

This book will help you become confident and prepared to live a happy and well-nourished life despite being a diabetic. Start your journey now!

Also, before you get started, I recommend you **joining our email newsletter** to receive updates on any upcoming new book releases or promotions. You can sign-up for free, and as a bonus, you will receive a gift. Our "*Health & Fitness Mistakes You Don't Know You're Making*" book! This book has been written to demystify, expose the top do's and don'ts and to finally equip you with the information you need to get in the best shape of your life. Due to the overwhelming amount of misinformation and lies told by magazines and self-proclaimed "gurus," it's becoming harder and harder to get reliable information to get in shape. You will have to go through dozens of biased, unreliable, and untrustworthy sources to get your health & fitness information. Everything you need to help you has been broken down in this book for you to easily follow and to immediately get results to achieve your desired fitness goals in the shortest amount of time.

Once again, to join our free email newsletter and to receive a free copy of this valuable book, please visit the link and signup now: **www.effingopublishing.com/gift.**

PART ONE: BEFORE THE DIVE

Welcome to the FIRST part of the book. In this part, we will delve into the basics of diabetes. What is it? What are the types? What risks? The ABC. What to eat? The how should and the how much.

CHAPTER 1: UNDERSTANDING DIABETES

More and more people nowadays are diagnosed with diabetes. Before, most people who happen to have the disease are adults age 30 and above. However, today, it can strike anyone, regardless of status and place. What's even more alarming is that the increase is not just a couple of thousands. We are talking millions here. Recent statistics state that over 30 million citizens of the US are diabetes positive, and over 420 million all over the world.

Now, you may ask. What is diabetes in the first place? What makes it so dangerous?

Well, diabetes is a condition where the blood sugar levels of a person rise above the normal. It usually happens when the human body cannot fully utilize the insulin released by the pancreas to regulate the sugar levels. For a diabetes-free person, insulin regulates the sugar level and helps use the sugar for energy. However, if someone is diagnosed to be suffering from diabetes, that person cannot correctly perform this task, causing a rise in sugar concentration in the blood.

Type 1, Symptoms and Risk Factors

Diabetes can occur in two types: Type 1 and Type 2. The more severe type is Type 1. Type 1 diabetes is also known as Juvenile Diabetes because it usually hits children and adolescents. However, anyone can have type 1. This type is not shared, and often, 10% of diabetes patients have this.

In type 1 diabetes, the patient's body does not produce insulin at all. It causes the patient to be dependent on insulin medication. It usually results as an effect of the immune system attacking the body's insulin-producing cells located in the pancreas. The attack usually ends up with the inability to produce insulin. Because there is no more insulin, the sugar in the blood cannot be processed, and it builds up, starving the cells of the energy required.

It often affects not just the blood but can also lead to problems with the eyes, nerves, heart, kidneys, and more. If left untreated, it can lead to death. Patients with Type 1 will have to rely on insulin therapy, possibly in their lifetime.

Symptoms

Here are some of the observable signs from a patient with Type 1 diabetes:

1. Frequent urination (bed-wetting for children)

2. Increased thirst

3. Rapid weight loss

4. Severe hunger

5. Fatigue

6. Irritability

7. Blurred vision

8. Dizziness and vomiting

9. Abdominal pain

10. Bad breath

11. Itchy skin

Risk Factors

There are a lot of factors that can affect the onset and progression of Type 1 diabetes. Here are some of the most prominent:

1. Genetics and family history

2. Food and eating habit

3. Stress

4. Geographic location

5. Environmental factors

6. General health

7. Age

Type 2, Symptoms and Risk Factors

Unlike Type 1 diabetes, Type 2 is more common. Approximately about 90% of diabetes patients have this. Compared also to type 1, type 2 does not rely too much on insulin therapy. People who usually have this are adults; that's why it is also called Adult Onset Diabetes. Although, more and more children are getting diagnosed with this.

People diagnosed to have type 2 diabetes still can produce insulin but not enough. And most of the time, though the body can create insulin, the body cannot recognize its use as it resists. It is called insulin resistance.

Treatments for this type is mostly on how to counter insulin resistance and to improve the production of insulin. These treatments primarily focus on proper diet, weight management, and having an active lifestyle. The only time there is medication when the sugar level is no longer manageable that it needs help with medication.

Symptoms

The symptoms that a person with type 2 diabetes may observe are similar to the symptoms of those with type 1. The only difference is that for type 2 diabetes patients, the onset of those symptoms is slower and less severe. Now, although the signs are not shouting diabetes, it is also the reason why they are mistaken for something else, such as signs of aging or stress. Hence, most people tend to overlook them.

Risk Factors

Like Type 1 diabetes, several factors can also trigger Type 2 diabetes. These factors include:

1. Genetics and family history

2. Food and eating habits

3. Lifestyle

4. Weight

5. Stress

6. High Blood Pressure

7. Hormonal problems

What to Do Pre-Diabetes?

Diabetes prevention is always better than treating it upon onset. Preventing diabetes is also quite easy though it needs commitment. It revolves around keeping a healthy lifestyle and avoiding health complications. The American Diabetes Association presents these simple steps to help prevent diabetes along with additional points:

1. **Become more active**

   One way of making sure that you don't develop diabetes is by keeping yourself busy. Engage in exercises and other physical activities to stimulate the metabolism of sugar. It is recommended to include aerobic exercise as well as resistance and endurance training as they have been proven to help prevent or control diabetes.

2. **Eat more fiber**

   Fiber brings many benefits to the body. It can help lower the risk of developing heart diseases. It can boost weight loss by increasing satiety. It can also help regulate your blood sugar levels. Fiber-rich foods are mostly vegetables, fruits, legumes and beans, nuts, and whole grains.

3. **Eat whole grains**

Instead of going for flour bread, go for whole-grains and other products instead. Aside from being evident as a source of fiber, whole grains are also to help curb your hunger, so you are less likely to keep on eating carbohydrates to sate your appetite. Thus, the next you want to eat some carbs, go for whole-grain foods like cereals, oats, pasta, etc.

4. **Lose weight**

Your weight can affect the onset of diabetes. If you are overweight or obese, you have a higher risk of developing diabetes. You need to lose those extra pounds to ensure a lesser risk. A study observed overweight participants who lost weight and found out that weight loss decreased their diabetes risk by 60%.

5. Healthy meals over diet

The primary purpose of diet fads is to help you lose weight. Although they can be useful in meeting that demand, they may not be sustainable when it comes to preventing diabetes in the long run. Hence, instead of focusing on dieting, why not focus on keeping your meals healthy instead?

6. Sleep well

Sleep is an essential aspect of health. If you wish to maintain good health, then you need to maintain a good sleeping habit. Chronic lack of sleep is correlated by some studies to lead to a higher risk of diabetes development.

7. Stay hydrated

Another key to keeping yourself at a lower risk for diabetes is to keep yourself well-hydrated and stick to water. Carbonated drinks and sugar-filled beverages will only put you at risk.

What to Do Upon Diagnosis?

Being diagnosed with diabetes is not easy. However, it does not spell the end of your world either. You can continue living as you are with some changes mixed in to help control your diabetes.

1. Exercise daily

Just like how to prevent diabetes, exercise also plays a vital role in controlling your diabetes. Exercise can help stimulate the production of insulin as well as your body's ability to utilize it well.

You don't have to start in a rush. Start with simple exercises and build your way. Small walks 30 min every morning is a good start. You can work your way up and add in more activities or increase the level.

2. Keep a healthy diet

Keep your meals healthy. Stick to non-starchy foods like asparagus, cucumber, carrots, salad greens, and tomato. Don't forget to settle for lean meats only. Some non-fat dairy products, lean poultry, fish, sweet potatoes, beans, and fruits. If you want to get some carbs in, keep it whole grain like brown rice, popcorn, quinoa, whole oats, and sorghum. Also, make sure to keep yourself well-hydrated with water.

3. Reduce stress

Stress can contribute to many diseases and conditions. Diabetes is no exception. Stress can raise your sugar levels and insulin resistance. Lower down the pressure by finding time to relax and managing the things that are potential causes of stress properly.

4. Quit your vices

Smoking and drinking liquor two vices that you should quit. Smoking and drinking too much alcohol can cause several problems aside from diabetes, such as respiratory and liver problems. Drinking alcohol can drop your sugar level since your liver will have to focus on ridding your blood of liquor rather than regulate your sugar levels.

5. Track everything

Do keep track of your daily living. Take of what you eat, drink, and do every day so you will quickly pick up unhealthy habits that you may develop that can trigger your diabetes more. If you are aiming to lose weight, this will especially helpful in keeping track of what you should and should not eat and drink.

6. Sleep well

Make sure to maintain a good sleeping routine. Having enough rest and sleep can do wonders for your body. Good sleep can boost your metabolism and other bodily functions, which is an essential aspect of controlling diabetes.

Mind the ABC

Whether you have diabetes or not, there are three things that you need to remember well. These will be your ABCs.

A is for A1C Test. With the A1C test, you can measure the level of your blood sugar within three months. It is usually used to diagnose if a person has Type 2 diabetes or not. It is recommended to at least have this test twice a year. Your goal to pass the test is to get a percent below 5.7. If you get a reading of 5.7 to 6.4, then you will be diagnosed as prediabetic. A reading of 6.5 and above percent means you have diabetes.

B is of Blood Pressure. Your blood pressure can have a significant impact on your diabetes. It is also one of the main things that can help determine your status. Your blood pressure is measured to know the rate at which your heart needs to work so it can keep your blood circulating. For diabetes patients, the blood pressure should be of utmost 130/80.

C is for Cholesterol. Cholesterol is the fat that is in your blood. It can build up in your arteries and form plaque, which damages arteries and inhibits blood flow. The body has two kinds, the LDL or Low-Density Lipoprotein and HDL or High-Density Lipoprotein. LDL is the "bad" cholesterol and should be below 100 mg/dl. However, a reading of 100-129 mg/dl can still be considered close to the ideal measurement, while 130-159 mg/dl is considered borderline. HDL is the "good" cholesterol.

Men are advised to have HDL above 40 mg/dl and women at above 50 mg/dl. The total amount of triglycerides should be the utmost at 200 mg/dl.

Make sure to keep up with your ABCs to ensure that you stay healthy and do not exacerbate things if youha diabetes.

Chapter 2: WHAT SHOULD YOU EAT?

Macronutrients are essential ingredients for good health. The body needs them for growth, proper metabolism, energy processing, and other vital functions. If you have type 2 diabetes, making sure to have these macronutrients have never been more critical.

There are three macronutrients that you need to have: carbohydrates, proteins, and fats. Carbohydrates have the most significant impact on your blood sugar, while proteins and fats, though they do not have a direct effect on your sugar levels, can still affect your overall health.

Carbohydrates

Carbohydrates are the body's primary energy source, and almost all foods contain carbohydrates. Because of its direct impact on the blood sugar levels, some call it the "great villain" for diabetics. However, that is not necessarily so.

There is no need to remove carbohydrates in your diet altogether because they are essential to the overall functioning of the body. What you need to do is to eliminate the bad carbohydrate sources and stick the healthy ones.

Fruits

Fruits can give you the fibers and carbohydrates as well as vitamins that you need. Compared to vegetables, fruits have higher carbohydrate-content. So, although healthy, they need to be eaten proportionally.

It is recommended to eat raw and fresh fruits than dried ones. But if you happen to buy canned ones. Make sure to check that there is no sugar added.

Vegetables

Vegetables are great heathy sources for carbs. They can be non-starchy or starchy. ***Non-starchy vegetables*** are low in calories but are high in fiber. They only contain a third of the carbs in fruits and starchy veggies. These are mostly green leafy vegetables such as broccoli, cauliflower, asparagus, artichokes, and other vegetables like tomatoes, eggplants, and peppers.

In eating non-starchy vegetables, there should be variety to get as many different nutrients and minerals. Stay away from canned and processed vegetables and stick to fresh produce. If canned veggies are unavoidable, make sure to select those with low sodium.

Starchy vegetables, on the other hand, contain more carbohydrates than non-starchy ones. Examples of these veggies are squash, peas, corn, and potatoes. They are good sources of vitamins, fibers, and minerals. But since they have more carbohydrates, they should be taken in smaller amounts than the non-starchy ones.

Grains and Beans

Grains and beans are also excellent sources of carbs. Grains have more carbohydrates than fruits, vegetables, and legumes. Grains can be refined or whole. Refined grains are those that have been processed already, to remove the bran and germs. They have lower fiber and nutrient content than whole grains. Whole grains are a healthier variety since they have more fibers and nutrients. For diabetic patients, whole grains are great meal choices. Beans and lentils are excellent sources of protein and high fibers and carbohydrates, although fewer than the others.

Proteins

Proteins are mainly for structural, hormonal, immune, and metabolic functions of the body. Proteins also provide more satisfaction and satiety during meals. Proteins are mostly from meat, poultry, eggs, fish, and seafood. Soy products like tofu and legumes are also excellent protein sources.

For meals, it is better to choose fish and seafood in your meals rather than red meat. If you want to have red meat, stick to the lean and skinless ones as they have less fat and cholesterol content. You need to avoid processed meats such as hot dogs, salami, luncheon meats, and more.

It is also recommended to spread out the consumption of meat in little portions throughout the day rather than eating a large quantity in a single meal. Studies show that the body can process protein better this way.

Fats

Fats are essential components for cell maintenance and the absorption of vitamins. They also provide more prolonged satiety during meals as they take longer to digest. They also offer a more concentrated source of energy though it takes longer to process.

Fats can either be saturated or unsaturated. Saturated fats are those that tend to stay solid at room temperatures such as margarine, butter, lard, animal fat, chicken skin, and processed snacks. Unsaturated fats are those that remain liquid at room temperature. Unsaturated fats are healthier and can be monounsaturated or polyunsaturated. Monounsaturated fats are in olive oil, nuts, and avocadoes. Polyunsaturated fats can a in fish rich in omega-3 such as salmon, sardines, tuna, mackerel, and oysters. Nuts like walnuts and flaxseed are also rich in these.

You must avoid saturated fats and load on unsaturated ones, especially omega-3, which is good for your heart.

Sodium

Although sodium is not a macronutrient, it is still a necessary component of the food that we eat. It can is in the majority of foods that we eat. It is because salt adds flavor to the food to make it more delicious and satisfying to eat. It is also a vital electrolyte source for the body, which is essential for the muscles and nerves.

Now, although there is no direct link between diabetes and sodium, it is still essential to keep the proper levels. Too much sodium can increase the risk of heart diseases. If you are at risk of heart diseases, then it will have adverse effects if you diagnosed with diabetes. It is recommended to keep sodium levels optimally at 2300 mg per day. It is for both people with or without diabetes.

Make sure to have the proper nutrients necessary for you to survive. Just make sure to keep these nutrients and minerals are appropriate and recommended levels. If you happen to exceed the recommended level, it can harm your health. Do keep up with the necessary tests, a healthy diet, and a healthier lifestyle to keep them at bay.

Chapter 3: HOW SHOULD YOU EAT?

For this chapter, we will be talking about the importance of knowing how much you should eat. It is not only essential to keep tabs of WHAT YOU EAT, but HOW MUCH YOU EAT as well. There two ways on how you can monitor how much you eat. The first one is by keeping tabs on your plate portion, and the second is counting your carbs.

Mind the Plate Portion

The first method you can use to monitor your meals and how much you consume is the plating or portioning method. This method is for those who do not have the time to keep up with more advanced carbohydrates and calorie tracking. Portioning is more relaxed as you do not have to count how many calories the food you eat have. In this method, you have to divide your plate into three portions of vegetables, protein, and carbohydrates.

Vegetables - ½ of the plate

Proteins - ¼ of the plate

Carbohydrates - ¼ of the plate.

For the vegetables, make sure to stick to the non-starchy veggies. Proteins should be fish, lean meat, poultry with no skin, eggs, nuts, or tofu. Your carbohydrates should be whole grain bread pasta, potato, corn, peas, or beans.

You can choose a small dessert bowl and add a serving of fresh fruits or low-fat yogurt. Stick to low-calorie drinks like tea or black coffee. Or, better yet, stick to water.

Count the Carbs

Once you have mastered the plating or portioning method, you can level up your meal monitoring and proceed to count your carbohydrates. In this method, you count the carbs you consume by grams for each meal, including snacks.

For men: It is recommended to keep carbohydrates at a max of 60 grams per meal, while snacks should be at a max of 30 grams.

For women: It is recommended to keep carbohydrates at 45 grams per meal and 15 grams for snacks.

Note: If you want to lose weight, you need to eat less the given amounts above.

For this method, you must know the meal portion for each recommended grams of carbohydrates. Below are some of the average carbohydrate gram count and their corresponding meal portion samples.

15 grams of carbs per serving

Grains

- 1 regular slice regular bread or 2 slices diet bread

- 1/3 cup of cooked pasta, rice, or quinoa

- ¾ cup of cold cereal or ½ cup of cooked cereal

- 1 flour tortilla at 6 inches

- 1/3 cup of brown rice

- ½ cup of cooked oatmeal

Starchy vegetables and legumes

- ½ cup of sweet potato

- ½ medium-sized potato

- ½ cup of plantain

- 1 small corn ear

- ½ cup corn, beans, lentils, peas

- 1 cup of squash (winter)

- ½ cup lentil soup

Non-starchy vegetables

- ½ cup of cooked veggies

- 1 cup of raw veggies

Fruits

- ½ grapefruit

- ½ medium-sized banana

- 1 small apple, pear, peach or orange

- 12 pieces of cherries or grapes

- ½ cup of frozen fruits, unsweetened

- ½ melon

- 1 cup of blackberries

- ¾ cup of blueberries

- 1 1/3 cup of strawberries

Sweeteners and Common snacks

- 1 tablespoon of honey, maple syrup, jelly

- 3 cups of popcorn

- 10-12 pieces of baked potato chips

- ¾ ounce of pretzels or crackers

Dairy products

- 8 ounces of cow's milk

- 8 ounces unsweetened soy milk

- 6 ounces plain unsweetened yogurt

- 6 ounces of Greek yogurt

These are just average measurements. Some of these measurements may vary, especially for sweeteners and snacks. It is recommended to always check the nutritional labels at the back of the containers for each food you plan to eat for more accuracy.

Chapter 4: HOW MUCH SHOULD YOU EAT?

The meals that you eat is usually based on a specific calorie count each day. This calorie count also depends on your height, age, weight, activity level, and whether you want to lose weight or maintain your current weight.

To Maintain a Healthy Weight

To maintain the current weight, men needs around 1800-2300 calories per day, while women need around 1700-2000 calories per day. These are only average calorie counts. If you want to know your calorie count, here are some straightforward calculations to do:

Sedentary lifestyle (little to no activity)

If you live a sedentary lifestyle and slightly overweight, the number of calories you need a day is at least 10 calories per pound.

Moderately active (walking about 1.5-3 miles a day)

If you take walks to up to 3 miles a day, then you are moderately active. Base your calorie count to 13 calories per pound.

Active (walking at least 3 miles a day), overweight

If you are busy and can walk more than 3 miles every day, then your calorie count will be based on 15 calories per pound.

To Lose the Extra Pounds

To lose weight, mean should have a daily calorie count of 1500-1800 while women must stick to 1200-1500. Generally, if you want to lose at least 1 pound per week, then you need to cut 500 calories from your daily calorie count. If you're going to lose 2 pounds per week, then cut your calories by 1000. Do take note though that cutting 1000 calories from your daily calorie count may have adverse effects on your health. Only do the 1000-calorie cut when you are physically capable of doing so.

The measurements stated above are only a standard average. The calorie counts may vary from person to person. To get a more accurate calorie count, you can use online calorie calculators. Better yet, you can ask experts, so you know how to proceed.

PART TWO: THE PLAN

Suddenly changing your diet is not easy. It may take months, even years, to build yourself up. However, to make that transition more comfortable for you, we have prepared a sample shopping list and a sample two-week meal plan that you can follow.

Chapter 5:PREPARATION AND SHOPPING

Preparation is crucial in any plan or change. For a Type 2 newly diagnosed diabetic, even for those who are not, prepping the kitchen as well as the possible things to buy is essential. Hence, for this chapter, we have outlined a preparation scheme that you can follow for your kitchen as well as a sample shopping list for the first two weeks of your journey. The ingredients of the shopping list include the ingredients for the meals included in the two-week plan in the following chapter.

Prepping the Kitchen

Having healthy ingredients is essential for any meal, be it for a diabetic patient or not. Hence, it is vital that before start planning your meals, you keep your ingredients stock up your kitchen with only healthy ingredients. But before you do that, you must clear out the tempting unhealthy and not-so-healthy foods first. These include high-sugar cereals, cookies, carbonated drinks like soda, ice cream, junk food, and other similar snacks. You also need to check the labels at the back and keep as little as possible of processed foods.

Once you have cleared out your kitchen, then you can stock up on these essential healthy ingredients. The following examples are only the most common must-haves in a healthy kitchen. You can choose to add or remove some of the items to suit your taste better.

PANTRY

Of all parts of the kitchen, the pantry is the most prone to get stocked with different foods and drinks. Hence, before you go on your next grocery shopping for what to place here, take a look at the following sample pantry contents first:

- Steel-cut oatmeal
- Vinegar

- Chia seeds
- Jam and jelly (low-sugar)

- Ground flaxseed
- Peanut butter (low-sodium)

- Plain unsalted nuts
- Tomato paste

- Whole-grain bread
- Whole-grain cereal

- Whole-grain crackers
- Whole-grain brown rice

- Whole-grain pasta
- Whole-grain quinoa

- Whole-grain tortillas
- Whole-grain barley

- Tomato sauce

- Beans and lentils (low-sodium)

- Tomatoes (canned, low-sodium)

- Vegetable oil (olive oil, canola oil)

- Tuna or salmon (canned, in water)

- Nonstick cooking spray

- Sweet potatoes

- Broth (canned, low-sodium)

Note: Make sure to look for at least 2 g of fiber per serving in the whole-grains you will buy.

FREEZER

You should also keep in mind not to get carried away in stocking up your fridge, especially with fatty meats and processed frozen goods. Here some contents you can include:

- Lean cut pork or tenderloin

- Fish (tuna, salmon, etc.)

- Skinless chicken or turkey

- Other seafood (stay alert for allergies)

- Lean beef

- Edamame

- Frozen meals

Note: Be sure to keep frozen meals at 400 calories or less with max 500 mg sodium, max 45 g carbohydrates, at least 6 g of fiber, and at least 15 g protein.

REFRIGERATOR

The next thing you to keep watch on is the refrigerator. It is prone to stocking with too many sweets and other similar carbohydrates. Here are some of what your fridge should have:

- Eggs

- Vegan protein (tofu, tempeh or seitan)

- Fresh fruits

- Dijon mustard

- Non-starchy vegetables

- Non-dairy milk (almond, coconut, soy)

- Low-calorie drinks (Ex. Seltzer)

- Non-fat milk

- Vegetable juice (Low-sodium)

- Non-fat yogurt (Ex. Greek yogurt)

- Low-fat cheese (parmesan, etc.)

MISCELLANEOUS

Here are other things you can stock up on, especially as additional flavor boosters for your meals. It is better to stick to these flavor enhancers as they have lower sodium, sugar, and calorie content than the typical ones used in a regular kitchen.

- Flavored vinegar (raspberry, etc.)

- Lemon or lime juice

- Low-sodium or no-sodium seasonings

- Ginger	- Lemon or lime zest
- Garlic	- avocado-lemon salsa
- Onions	- Marinara sauce
- Low-sodium soy sauce	- Allspice
- Rosemary	- Parsley
- Cayenne pepper	- Black pepper
- Basil	- Oregano

- Cumin   - Pepper flakes

- Thyme

SOME EQUIPMENT YOU MAY NEED

Aside from the ingredients mentioned above, having the right equipment in your kitchen will also make prepping up the meals healthier. Here some of the essentials:

- Kitchen scale   - Measuring cups or spoons

- Blender   - Food processor

- Spiralizer (Vegetable)   - Steamer

Basic Shopping List

Before we delve into the actual sample meal plans, we have presented here a sample shopping list for you. The contents of this shopping list are all the most common healthy ingredients that are typical components of healthy meals for diabetic and non-diabetic patients.

Meat

- Ground turkey
- Chicken breast, skinless
- Boneless pork, top loin
- Flank steak

Seafood

- Tilapia fillets
- Scallops
- Sole fillets
- Halibut

Dairy or Alternatives and Eggs

- Butter
- Feta cheese
- Milk, almond or skim
- Cottage cheese
- Goat cheese
- Greek yogurt

Produce

- Avocado
- Banana
- Chives
- English cucumbers
- Garlic
- Cauliflower
- Lettuce
- Limes
- Mushrooms
- Habanero peppers
- Apple
- Eggplant
- Corn kernels
- Fennel bulbs
- Carrots
- Broccoli
- Green beans
- Mint
- Red bell peppers
- Red and sweet onions

- Scallions
- Tomatoes
- Kale
- Thyme
- Parsley
- Strawberries
- Spinach
- Zucchini
- Basil
- Oregano
- Blueberries
- Raspberries

Bottled or Canned Items

- Chicken broth (low-sodium)

- Vegetable broth (sodium-free)

- Olive oil, extra virgin

- Nonstick cooking spray

- Dijon mustard

- Navy items

- Chickpeas (sodium-free)

- Worcestershire sauce

- Healthy Pumpkin puree

- Unsweetened applesauce

- Sun-dried tomatoes

Pantry Items

- Flour, whole-wheat	- Pitas, whole-wheat
- Bread, whole-wheat	- Tortilla wraps, whole-wheat
- Bun, whole-wheat	- Couscous, whole-wheat
- Almond flour	- Linguine, whole-wheat
- Baking powder	- Pistachios
- Baking soda	- Almond, chopped
- Balsamic vinegar	- Pine nuts
- Sea salt	- Ground cinnamon
- Paprika	- Honey
- Vanilla extract	- Granulated sweetener

- Ground cumin   - Black pepper

- Garlic powder   - Chili powder

- Ground coriander   - Bread crumbs

- Quinoa   - Oats

- Coffee beans   - Pecans

- Bulgur wheat   - Apple cider vinegar

- Stevia

You can choose to add more to the shopping list above in case you have more things that you need. Just remember to always check the labels at the back for canned and bottled items. Always select those that have low-sodium or no sodium content. For produce, always go for the fresh if you can or go for raw dried ones if fresh produce is not readily available.

Chapter 6: the TWO-WEEK PLAN

You have prepped your kitchen as well as done your shopping. Now, what's next?

Well, start preparing meals, of course! But we understand that it may be confusing at first on how to choose which meals to prepare. So, we have taken it upon ourselves to provide a sample meal plan that you can follow for two weeks. All the meals mentioned here have recipes and prepping instructions that you can follow in the next chapter.

These are all delicious and healthy meals that can help you settle your first two weeks of changing your lifestyle for the batter after being a newly diagnosed type 2 diabetic.

Week 1 Meal Plan

Monday

Breakfast: Blueberry Lemon Muffins

Lunch: Chicken Stew, Whole-wheat Couscous with Pecans

Dinner: Baked Honey-Dijon Chops, and Quinoa Vegetable Skillet

Tuesday

Breakfast: Tasty Chia Pudding

Lunch: Blue Cheese Chicken Burger, and Home-made kale chips

Dinner: Spicy Sole Fillet, and Zucchini Strips in Creamy Avocado Pesto

Wednesday

Breakfast: Mushroom Frittata with Goat Cheese

Lunch: Tilapia with Creamy Cucumber Sauce, and Fennel and Chickpeas

Dinner: Mediterranean Steak Sandwich

Thursday

Breakfast: Whipped Almond Cottage Cheese with Banana

Lunch: Pork Chop Diane, and Baked Eggplant with Goat Cheese

Dinner: Sweet Potato Caribbean Chicken, Home-made Kale Chips

Friday

Breakfast: Healthy Pumpkin Apple Waffles

Lunch: Tilapia with Creamy Cucumber Sauce, and Fennel and Chickpeas

Dinner: Wheat Bun Turkey Burger, and Baked Eggplant with Goat Cheese

Saturday

Breakfast: Mushroom Frittata with Goat Cheese

Lunch: Blue Cheese Chicken Burger, and Home-made kale chips

Dinner: Herb-crusted Halibut and Whole-wheat Couscous with Pecans

Sunday

Breakfast: Supreme Veggie Scramble

Lunch: Chicken Stew, Whole-wheat Couscous with Pecans

Dinner: Tilapia with Creamy Cucumber Sauce, and Fennel and Chickpeas

Week 2 Meal Plan

Monday

Breakfast: Whipped Almond Cottage Cheese with Banana

Lunch: Pork Chop Diane, and Quinoa Vegetable Skillet

Dinner: Spicy Sole Fillet, and Zucchini Strips in Creamy Avocado Pesto

Tuesday

Breakfast: Supreme Veggie Scramble

Lunch: Herb-crusted Halibut, and Whole-wheat Couscous with Pecans

Dinner: Coffee-Marinated Steak, and Quinoa Vegetable Skillet

Wednesday

Breakfast: Tasty Chia Pudding

Lunch: Chicken Stew, Home-made Kale Chips

Dinner: Pork Chop Diane, and Zucchini Strips in Creamy Avocado Pesto

Thursday

Breakfast: Mushroom Frittata with Goat Cheese

Lunch: Coffee-Marinated Steak, and Quinoa Vegetable Skillet

Dinner: Herb-crusted Halibut, and Whole-wheat Couscous with Pecans

Friday

Breakfast: Whipped Almond Cottage Cheese with Banana

Lunch: Baked Honey-Dijon Chops, Baked Eggplant with Goat Cheese

Dinner: Chicken Stew, and Whole-wheat Couscous with Pecans

Saturday

Breakfast: Blueberry Lemon Muffins

Lunch: Scallops in Orange, and Home-made Kale Chips

Dinner: Wheat Bun Turkey Burger, and Baked Eggplant with Goat Cheese

Sunday

Breakfast: Healthy Pumpkin Apple Waffles

Lunch: Coffee-Marinated Steak, and Quinoa Vegetable Skillet

Dinner: Spicy Sole Fillet, and Baked Eggplant with Goat Cheese

The meals included in the plan above can easily be interchanged depending on your preference and taste. However, for meals, you do not group abundant protein sources on the same day to disperse these sources throughout the day. For example, having breakfast with a chicken meal, then lunch with lamb or pork, then dinner with beef. The body is said to digest better and process these sources gradually and not in a single seating.

PART THREE: THE SCRUMPTIOUS RECIPE

It is essential that cooking your meals instead of eating take out it is vital to keep yourself healthy despite being a diabetic. That is why in this chapter, you will find the recipes of the meals included in the sample two-week plan as well as some additional examples. The recipes here have been categorized as breakfast meals, pork and beef, poultry, fish and seafood, veggies, and smoothies for easier access.

Chapter 7: BREAKFAST

Breakfast is the most important meal of the day. However, sometimes, because of the hectic schedule, most people miss breakfast. Well, with the recipes below, you will never miss breakfast again. They are all fast and easy to make so that you will have your breakfast in minutes.

Tasty Chia Pudding

Ingredients

- 3 tbsp chia seeds
- 1 cup milk, low-fat (coconut or almond)
- ½ tbsp honey or stevia
- ¼ tsp vanilla

Procedure

1. In a bowl, mix the chia seeds, honey, vanilla, and milk. Let it sit for 5 minutes then stir again until no more clumps are left.

2. Transfer to a glass or mason jar and refrigerate for at least 2 hours or overnight.

Total Calories:237 calories per serving

Whipped Almond Cottage Cheese with Banana

Ingredients

- 3 8-oz. cottage cheese, low-fat or non-fat
- 4 tbsp almond butter
- 2 large bananas, sliced

Procedure

1. Blend the cottage cheese and almond butter until smooth. Then, divide into 4 bowls. Top with sliced bananas.

2. You can also add almond nuts.

Total Calories:270 calories per serving

Lemon Blueberry Muffin

Ingredients

- 1 cup fresh blueberries

- ¾ cup sour cream

- 2 cups all-purpose flour

- 2 tsp baking powder

- ¼ tspbaking soda

- ¼ tsp sea salt

- ¼ cup lemon juice

- Lemon zest, 1 lemon

- 2 large eggs

- 2/3cup granulated sugar

- ½ cup unsalted butter, melted

Procedure

1. Preheat oven to 375°F.

2. In a large bowl, mix the baking powder, baking soda, flour, and salt. Add in the eggs, sour cream, lemon juice, lemon zest, sugar, and melted butter. Make sure to mix until thick and lumpy. Add in the blueberries. Stir.

3. Grease a 12-cup muffin pan and scoop equal amounts of the batter into each cup. Bake for 15-20 minutes or until no more comes off when you insert a toothpick. Cool and serve.

Total Calories:258 calories per serving

Healthy Pumpkin Apple Waffles

Ingredients

- 1 ¼ cup wholewheat flour
- 1 tbsp baking powder
- 1 tbspgranulated sugar
- ½ tsp salt

- ½ cup canned pumpkin puree

- 2 small apples, finely diced

- 1 egg

- 1 cup milk, low-fat

- 2 tbsp canola oil

- 2 tsp cinnamon

Procedure

1. Preheat the waffle iron or nonstick pan if there is no waffle iron.

2. In a bowl, mix the flour, baking powder, cinnamon, sugar, and salt. When combined well, add the milk, oil, egg, and pumpkin puree. Mix well, then add the diced apples.

3. Scoop about 1/3 cup and pour it into the waffle iron per cooking.

Total Calories:170 calories per serving

Mushroom Frittata with Goat Cheese

Ingredients

- 8 large eggs
- 4 oz. wild mushroom, sliced
- ½ cup milk, low-fat
- 3 oz. goat cheese, crumbled
- 3 tbsp olive oil or vegetable oil
- ¾ cup zucchini
- 1 large shallot, sliced
- 1 clove garlic, minced
- ¼ cup onion, chopped
- Salt and pepper

Procedure

1. Preheat oven to 350°F.

2. In a skillet, sauté the shallots and garlic in 1 tbsp of oil over medium-high heat. Add in the sliced mushrooms and sauté for 5-10 minutes, until the

mushrooms are a deep brown. Then, add the zucchini and sauté for another 2-3 minutes. Transfer to a plate and set aside.

3. Mix the eggs and milk and season with salt and pepper. Make sure to whisk until frothy.

4. Wipe clean the same skillet, then add 2 tbsp of oil. Swirl the skillet as you pour the egg mix to make a thin crust. Then, add the mushroom mixture and the crumbled goat cheese.

5. Transfer the pan into the oven and bake for 15-20 minutes or until cooked thoroughly. Slide the baked frittata and slice into wedges. Serve.

Total Calories:214 calories per serving

Chapter 8: pork and beef

Meat is an excellent source of protein. Hence, meals with lean meats are great additions to any meal. Here you will have a choice between pork and beef. Whichever your choice is, we have sample recipes on both that you can try out:

Pork Chop Diane

Ingredients

- 4 boneless pork chops (top loin, 1 inch thick)
- 1 tbsp water
- 1 tbsp butter
- 1 tbsp parsley or oregano
- 1 tbsp Worcestershire sauce
- 1 tsp lemon juice
- 1 tsp Dijon mustard
- 1 tsp lemon-pepper seasoning

Procedure

1. In a bowl, mix the Worcestershire sauce, water, Dijon mustard, and lemon juice. Then, set aside.

2. Clean the chops by trimming off the fat. Coat both sides with the lemon-pepper seasoning. Fry the pork chops with butter for 10-12 minutes over medium heat.

3. Heat the sauce on the same skillet and scrape in the crusty bits. Then, pour over the pork chops. Sprinkle with parsley and serve.

Total Calories:178 calories per serving per serving

Baked Honey-Dijon Chops

Ingredients

- 4 boneless pork chops, loin
- 1 tbsp honey
- 1 tbsp Dijon mustard
- Dash of black pepper

Procedure

1. Preheat the oven to 350-400°F.

2. Mix the honey and mustard then brush all over the pork chops. Sprinkle both sides with black pepper.

3. Place the chops on a baking pan and cover with foil. Bake for 30 minutes or until the internal pork temperature is at 145°F. Serve.

Total Calories:167 calories per serving

Mediterranean Steak Sandwich

Ingredients

- 4 think pork steaks
- 4 Whole-wheat bread
- 1 bag spinach
- 1 red onion, large, sliced
- 1 clove garlic, crushed
- 3 tbsp red wine
- 6 tbsp olive oil
- 1 ½ tsp oregano, dried
- ¾ cup Mediterranean feta cheese
- 6 slices fontina cheeses
- 1 ½ cup mozzarella, shredded
- 1 tsp onion powder
- 1 tsp garlic powder
- Dash of salt and pepper

Procedure

1. Preheat the oven to 375° F.

2. Brush the whole-wheat bread with olive oil and grill until grill marks appear. Set aside.

3. Season both sides of the steaks with the salt and pepper. Drizzle with wine and olive oil. Place in a baking dish, cover with foil and bake for 15-18 minutes or until cooked.

4. On a skillet, sauté the spinach and garlic until spinach wilts. Season with salt and pepper.

5. Assemble the sandwich: hoagie roll, steak, onions, spinach, feta cheese, fontina cheese, mozzarella. Bake again for 8-10 minutes or until cheese melts. Top with the remaining hoagie roll. Serve.

Total Calories:520 calories per serving

Coffee-Marinated Steak

Ingredients

- 2 lbs. beef sirloin steak, ¾ to 1-inch thick

- 2 tbsp Worcestershire sauce

- 2 tbsp vinegar

- 2 tbsp sesame seeds

- 4 cloves garlic, minced

- 1 onion, medium, chopped

- 1 cup of soy sauce

- 1 cup brewed black coffee

- 6 tbsp butter

Procedure

1. In a pan or skillet, sautéthe sesame seeds in butter. Then, add garlic and onion and continue sautéing until soft.

2. In a bowl, combine the soy sauce, coffee, vinegar, sesame mixture, and Worcestershire sauce. Pour half into a bowl, put in the steak, and marinate them overnight. Refrigerate the other half of the marinade.

3. Remove the steak from the marinade and grill for 8-10 minutes over medium heat. Warm the refrigerated marinade and serve with the steak.

Total Calories:307 calories per serving

Grilled Beef & Veggie Kebab

Ingredients

- 1 lb. sirloin steak, cut and trimmed, about 32 chunks
- 16 mushrooms, button
- 16 cherry tomatoes
- 1 bell pepper (green or red), cut into 16 pieces
- Large Onion, cut into 16 chunks, 1-inch
- ¾ cup balsamic vinegar
- ¾ cup olive oil
- 2 tbsp whole-grain or Dijon mustard
- 1 tbsp oregano
- 1 tbsp rosemary
- 2 cloves garlic, sliced
- ½ tsp sea salt
- ½ tsp ground black pepper

Procedure

1. In a small bowl, combine the balsamic vinegar, oregano, mustard, rosemary, garlic, black pepper, and salt. Set aside as marinade.

2. Alternately skewer the beef, bell pepper, mushrooms, onion, and tomatoes. You can choose your arrangement. Marinade the kebabs and refrigerate overnight.

3. Preheat the grill to medium heat. Grill the kebabs 10-15 minutes or until desired doneness. Serve

Total Calories:237 calories per serving

Chapter 9: poultry

If pork and beef are not your things, then perhaps poultry-based meals are the way to go. Here are a few notable recipes that you should try. What's even better is that they are all under 400 calories. Worth a try!

Chicken Stew

Ingredients

- 1 tbsp canola oil or olive oil
- ½ kg boneless chicken thighs, skinless, 1 ½ inch cuts
- 4 carrots, thinly sliced
- 2 cups carrots, sliced
- 1 cup celery, sliced
- 2/3 cup leeks, sliced
- 3 garlic cloves, minced
- 2 cups chicken broth, low-sodium
- ¾ cup red potato, cubed
- 1 cup green beans

- 2 tsp rosemary
- ½ cup milk, non-fat
- 1 tbsp flour
- ¼ tsp black pepper

Procedure

1. In a deep pan, combine the chicken, leeks, celery, carrots, and garlic. Sauté for a bit, then add the chicken. Cook for 8-10 minutes or until chicken is brown and the vegetables are soft. Add in the potatoes, rosemary, beans, and black pepper. Add the broth and boil under medium heat. Then, reduce the heat and simmer for 20-25 minutes.

2. In a separate bowl, mix the flour and the milk. Mix well, then add to the stew. Boil for 2 minutes or until the stew thickens. Then, serve.

Total Calories: 269calories per serving

Sweet Potato Caribbean Chicken

Ingredients

- ½ kg sweet potato, peeled and shredded
- 4 boneless chicken breasts, skinless, halved
- 4 tbsp water
- 1 egg
- 1 tbsp olive oil
- ¼ tsp sea salt
- 1/4 tsp black pepper
- 1 tsp Jamaican jerk seasoning (sodium-free)
- ¼ cup flour
- Avocado-mango salsa
- Dash of cayenne pepper
- Nonstick cooking spray

Procedure

1. Place the sweet potatoes on a microwave-safe container. Add 2 tbsp of water then cover with cling wrap. Microwave over medium temperature for 8-10 minutes. Drain off the water then set aside.

2. In a bowl, combine the egg, 2 tbsp water, ¼ tsp salt, 1/8 tsp black pepper, flour. Mix well. Add in the sweet potatoes and make sure to coat them thoroughly.

3. On a skillet, scoop about ¼ cup of the mixture and fry for 4-5 minutes. It makes about eight cakes.

4. On a separate bowl, mix the seasoning, remaining salt, black pepper, and cayenne pepper. Coat the chicken breasts evenly on each half.

5. Grill the chickens over medium heat for 10-12 minutes. Slice thinly once cooked well.

6. Serve the chicken with the salsa and sweet potato cake.

Total Calories:387calories per serving

Wheat Bun Turkey Burger

Ingredients

- 1 large egg
- 1 ¼ lb. lean turkey, ground
- 6 whole-wheat buns
- 2/3cup soft whole wheat bread crumbs
- ½ cup celery, chopped

- 1/4 cup onion, chopped
- 1 tbsp parsley, minced
- 1 tsp Worcestershire sauce
- 1 tsp oregano, dried
- ½ tsp sea salt
- ¼ tsp black pepper

Procedure

1. In a bowl, mix the egg, celery, onion, bread crumbs, parsley, Worcestershire sauce, salt, and black pepper. Add the ground turkey and mix well. Form 6 patties.

2. Grill or fry the patties until cooked or until juices run clear. Serve on buns. You can choose to add lettuce, tomatoes, etc.

Total Calories:293 calories per serving

Blue Cheese Chicken Burger

Ingredients

- 1 onion, medium, chopped
- 1 egg
- 3 tbsp dry bread crumbs
- 2 tbsp blue cheese, crumbled
- 1 clove garlic, minced
- 2 tsp Dijon mustard
- ¼ tsp black pepper

- 12 ounces chicken breast, ground
- 4 tsp olive oil
- 4 whole-wheat burger buns
- 2 tbsp low-fat blue cheese dressing (optional)
- 4 slices tomato
- 4 lettuce leaves

Procedure

1. In a bowl, combine the bread crumbs, egg, blue cheese, garlic, pepper, chopped onions, and ground chicken breast. Mix well.

2. Shape the mixture into patties about ¾ inch thick.

3. Add olive oil to the pan then fry the patties over medium heat for 15-18 minutes. Don't forget to turn the patties to avoid burning.

4. Split the buns into halves. Layer the burger as you want, or you can follow the order from bottom to top: bun, patty, salad dressing, lettuce, tomato, bun.

Total Calories:341calories per serving

Lemon Chicken

Ingredients

- 4 boneless chicken breasts, skinless
- 1 tbsp olive oil
- Lemon juice (1 lemon)
- ½ tsp onion powder
- ½ tsp white pepper
- 1 ½ tsp oregano, fresh
- Nonstick cooking spray

Procedure

1. Preheat oven to 375°F.

2. Divide an aluminum foil into 4 packets and spray with nonstick cooking spray. Place a chicken on each foil.

3. Drizzle the chickens with olive oil and lemon juice. Sprinkle the onion powder, oregano, and white pepper. Top with lemon zest. Seal the packets and bake for 30 minutes. Serve.

Total Calories:195 calories per serving

CHAPTER 10: FISH AND SEAFOOD

Fish and seafood are some of the healthiest ingredients you can have in your meals. Don't just cook up pork, beef, or poultry-based meals. Add in some delicious fish or seafood recipes too. Hence, you should not miss out on these easy and yummy recipes.

Tilapia with Creamy Cucumber Sauce

Ingredients

- 4 tilapia fish fillets
- 2/3 cup whole-wheat flour
- 1 lemon, cut in half (zest and garnish)
- 1 tbsp butter
- ¼ tsp paprika
- ¼ tsp pepper
- ½ tsp kosher salt or sea salt
- 1 English cucumber, cut lengthwise

- 2 shallots, thinly sliced

- 2 tbsp capers

- 1 cup sour cream or Greek yogurt

- 3 tbsp white wine

- 2 tbsp dill, minced

- Salt, pepper, cayenne pepper

Procedure

1. In a bowl, combine the flour, paprika, salt, pepper, cayenne, and lemon zest.

2. Coat the fish fillets with the flour mixture and fry in butter over medium heat for 3-4 minutes. Plate and squeeze half of the lemon over the fillets.

3. On a separate pan, sauté the shallots in white wine and simmer over medium heat for about 2 minutes. Add in the cucumber and capers, and simmer until cucumber is warm. Add in the sour cream or Greek yogurt, dill, salt, and black pepper and sauté for 2 more minutes. Serve the fish fillets and drizzle with the sauce.

Total Calories:357 calories per serving

Spicy Sole Fillet

Ingredients

- 1lb. sole fillet
- ¼ cup low-fat milk
- ¼ cup all-purpose flour
- 1 tsp black pepper
- 1 tsp cayenne
- 1 tsp paprika
- 1 tsp thyme
- 1 tsp sea salt
- 1 tsp olive oil

Procedure

1. In a bowl, soak the sole fillets in milk for 12-15 minutes. Set aside.

2. In a separate bowl, mix the flour, pepper, cayenne, paprika, thyme, and salt. Coat the fillets with the powder mixture and fry in olive oil over medium heat for 2-3 minutes or until cooked. Serve.

Total Calories:270 calories per serving

Herb-Crusted Halibut

Ingredients

- 4 halibut fillets
- ¾ cup panko bread crumbs
- 1/3cup parsley, chopped
- ¼ cup dill, chopped
- ¼ cup chives, chopped
- 1 tsp olive oil
- 1 tsp lemon zest
- Salt and pepper

Procedure

1. Preheat the oven to 400 ° F.

2. In a large bowl, mix the bread crumbs, chives, olive oil, dill, parsley, lemon zest, salt, and pepper. Coat the halibut fillets with the crumb mixture.

3. Place the coated fillet in a baking dish and bake for 10-15 minutes or until crumbs are brown.

Total Calories:273 calories per serving

Scallops in Orange

Ingredients

- 4 tbsp peanut oil
- 1 ½ lb. scallops
- ½ cup of orange juice
- 1 tsp soy sauce
- ½ tsp grated orange zest
- 1 tspblack pepper
- 1 tsp salt
- 2 cloves garlic, minced

Procedure

1. Season the scallops with salt and pepper. Sauté in peanut oil over medium heat until brown and plate when done.

2. On the same skillet, sauté the minced garlic, soy sauce, orange juice, orange zest for 2-3 minutes or until sauce thickens.

3. Pour the orange sauce over the scallops and serve.

Total Calories:291 calories per serving

Grilled Fish with Lemon-Parsley Mix

Ingredients

- 6 fish fillets (any lean white fish)

- 6 tbsp yogurt-based margarine

- 3 lemons, divided into half

- 3 tbsp fresh parsley, chopped

- 1 tsp lemon zest

- ½ tsp sea salt

- ½ tsp dried rosemary

- Nonstick cooking spray

Procedure

1. In a bowl, mix the parsley, lemon zest, rosemary, yogurt-based margarine, and sea salt. Set aside.

2. Grill the fish for 2-3 minutes. Squeeze some lemon juice over each fillet and top with the parsley and margarine mixture. Serve.

Total Calories: 211 calories per serving

Chapter 11: veggies

Vegetables are even more a must than meats. You need vegetables to balance your nutritional intake. Hence, you should spend some time to learn some vegetable recipes too. Here are some great recipes to start with:

Supreme Veggie Scramble

Ingredients

- 6 eggs
- ¼ cup milk, low-fat
- ¼ cup chopped fresh tomato
- ¼ cup shredded Cheddar cheese
- ¼ cup olive oil
- ¼ cup sliced fresh mushrooms
- ¼ cup chopped onions
- ¼ cup chopped green bell peppers

Procedure

1. In a bowl, mix the eggs, milk, and tomatoes. Set aside.

2. In a skillet., fry the bell peppers, onions, and mushroom in olive oil over medium heat until onion appears transparent. Add in the egg mixture and sauté for 2 minutes. Add in the cheese and cook for another 1 minute. Serve.

Total Calories:182 calories per serving

Zucchini Strips in Creamy Avocado Pesto

Ingredients

- 1 avocado, ripe
- 3 zucchinis, cut into ¼ inch noodle strips
- 1 clove garlic
- ½ cup fresh basil
- 1 tbsp lemon juice
- 2 tbsp olive oil

- Water

- Salt and pepper

Procedure

1. Blend the avocado, basil, garlic, and lemon juice until smooth. Add 1 tbsp olive oil, water as needed, a pinch of salt and pepper. Continue blending sauce appears thick. Pour on a bowl and set aside.

2. In a pan, sauté the zucchini strips in remaining olive oil over medium heat for 3-5 minutes or until soft. Add into the sauce and serve.

Total Calories:362 calories per serving

Quinoa Vegetable Skillet

Ingredients

- 1 cup quinoa
- 2 cups broccoli, steamed
- 2 cups cherry tomatoes, sliced
- ½ cup craisins
- 1 sweet potato, chopped
- 2 cups butternut squash, chopped
- 2 cups vegetable stock
- ¼ cup lemon zest
- 1 tbsp lemon juice
- Salt and pepper

Procedure

1. On a deep pan, boil the vegetables over medium heat for 10-12 minutes or until tender. Drain the water and cook in a skillet with olive oil for 5-7 minutes or until tender. Season with salt and pepper. Set aside.

2. In a saucepan, cook the quinoa with chicken stock, lemon juice, and lemon zest for 15 minutes. Remove

from the heat and settle for 5 minutes. Then, open the lid and fluff the quinoa. Set aside.

3. On the same skillet as the vegetables, add the quinoa, tomatoes, and broccoli. Stir for 5 minutes. Add the craisins then season with salt and pepper. Serve, hot or cold.

Total Calories:274 calories per serving

Baked Eggplant with Goat Cheese

Ingredients

- 1 eggplant
- 4 oz. goat cheese softened
- 1 ½ cups panko bread crumbs, toasted
- 4 tbsp butter
- 1 egg white
- 1 large egg
- 1 cup marinara sauce
- 2 tbsp garlic, minced
- ½ cup fresh basil, chopped
- 1 tbsp kosher salt

Procedure

1. Preheat oven to 400 °F.

2. Slice the eggplants into 1-inch thick slices. Place the eggplants on a plate and sprinkle with salt to drain the bitterness. Set aside for 30 minutes. Then, rinse with water to remove the salt. Wipe dry and set aside.

3. In a skillet, sauté the garlic in butter over medium heat for about 1 minute.

4. On a large bowl, combine the toasted bread crumbs and garlic-butter mixture. Mix well then place on a baking pan with parchment 5-8 minutes or until golden browned. Transfer to a bowl when done.

5. In a small bowl, mix the egg white and whole egg — season with salt and pepper. Then, set aside.

6. Dip the eggplant slices into the egg mixture and then into the crumb mixture. Make sure to coat each slice thoroughly. Arrange the coated eggplants into the baking pan and bake for 20 minutes or until soft.

7. Remove the baking dish with eggplants from the oven. Top the eggplants with marinara sauce, goat cheese, and chopped basil. Bake again for another 10 minutes or until the cheese becomes golden brown. Serve.

Total Calories:201 calories per serving

Home-made Kale Chips

Ingredients

- 1 bunch kale
- 1 tbsp olive oil
- ¼ tsp black pepper
- 1/8 tsp kosher or sea salt
- 1/8 tsp garlic powder

Procedure

1. Preheat oven to 300 °F. Line the baking pans with parchment.

2. Wash and dry the kale leaves thoroughly. Tear the leaves enough to fill about 8 cups.

3. In a bowl, toss with leaves with salt, pepper, olive oil, and garlic powder. Bake the leaves for 20-25 minutes or until crisp. Cool then serve.

Total Calories:97calories per serving

Chapter 12: SMOOTHIE

If you don't like eating hard meals or are too much in a hurry to prep up a decent meal. Don't worry. You can always go for refreshing, healthy smoothies instead. They are healthy and so easy to make. You can also have them to-go and gobble them up while on the train or as you arrive at your desk. Try out the following simple smoothies:

Avocado Blueberry Banana Smoothie

Ingredients

- ½ cup almond milk
- ½ ripe avocado
- 1 banana
- 1 cup spinach
- 2 cups blueberries
- 1 tbsp ground flaxseed
- 1 tbsp almond butter
- ¼ tsp cinnamon

Procedure

1. Place all the wet ingredients inside a blender and blend. Then, add the solid ingredients and blend again until well-mixed and smooth. For a thicker finish, add ice. For a thinner finish, add more almond milk.

Total Calories:283 calories per serving

Strawberry Oats Smoothie

Ingredients

- 12-14 strawberries, sliced
- 1 banana, sliced
- ½ cup oats
- 1 cup almond milk
- 2 tbsp honey

Procedure

1. Blend the oats until they become finer. Then, add bananas, strawberries, almond milk, and honey. Blend until well-mixed and smooth. Add ice for a thicker consistency or add more almond milk for a thinner consistency.

Total Calories: 254 calories per serving

Nutty Banana Raspberry Smoothie

Ingredients

- 2 tbsp peanut butter, unsweetened

- 1 cup raspberries

- 1 large banana

- 1 cup almond milk

Procedure

1. Mix in all the ingredients in a blender. Blend for 10 minutes or until smooth then serve. Add ice to make it thicker then blend again. Add almond milk to make it thinner.

Total Calories:200calories per serving

Kale, Ginger and Strawberry Smoothie

Ingredients

- 6 pcs Kale leaves, fresh

- 2 tsp grated ginger

- 1 cup strawberries, fresh

- 2 tsp honey

- 3 tbsp lime juice

- ½ cup of water

- 1 cup ice cube

Procedure

1. Mix in all the ingredients in a blender. Blend for 10 minutes or until smooth then serve. Good for two servings.

Total Calories:205 calories per serving

Piney Kale Smoothie

Ingredients

- 1 cup Greek yogurt, plain
- 3 cups baby kale
- 1 cup cucumber
- 1 ½ cup pineapple cubes
- 2 tbsp hemp seeds

Procedure

1. Put all the ingredients into a blender and blend until you get your desired consistency or until smooth. Add some ice for more thickness or add ½ cup almond milk to make it slurry and thinner.

Total Calories:206 calories per serving

Conclusion

Indeed, being diagnosed with diabetes is not easy. A lot of things need to change in your lifestyle, especially the food that you eat. But it doesn't have to be tedious and overwhelming. Diabetes is not the end. It is merely a change that you will have to get accustomed to.

We hope that with this book, you can garner insights on how you will move on from your diagnoses and help yourself improve by applying the information you learned from this book. We also hope that the recipes we have included will provide you with not only readily-available meals but to inspire you to try your very own creations as well.

FINAL WORDS

Thank you again for purchasing this book!

We hope this book can help you.

The next step is for you to **join our email newsletter** to receive updates on any upcoming new book releases or promotions. You can sign-up for free, and as a bonus, you will also receive our "*7 Fitness Mistakes You Don't Know You're Making*" book! This bonus book breaks down many of the most common fitness mistakes and will demystify many of the complexities and science of getting into shape. Having all this fitness knowledge and science organized into an actionable step-by-step book will help you get started in the right direction in your fitness journey! To join our free email newsletter and grab your free book, please visit the link and signup: **www.effingopublishing.com/gift**

Finally, if you enjoyed this book, then we would like to ask you for a favor, would you be kind enough to leave a review for this book? It would be much appreciated! Thank you, and good luck on your journey!

ABOUT THE CO-AUTHORS

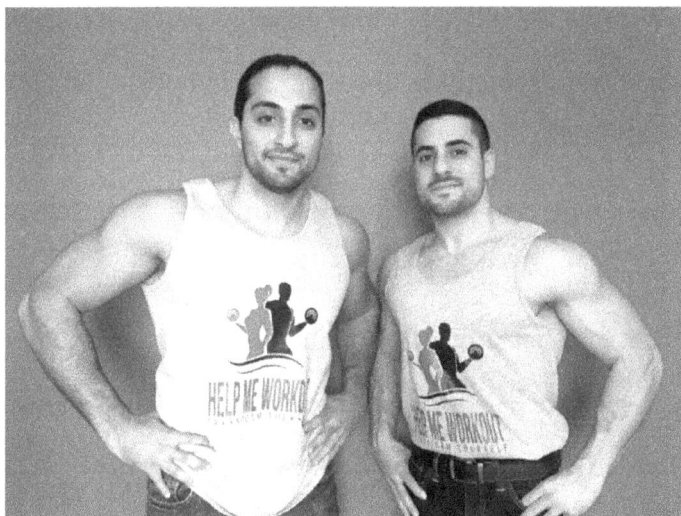

Our name is Alex & George Kaplo; we're both certified personal trainers from Montreal, Canada. We will start by saying we are not the biggest guys you will ever meet, and this has never really been our goal. We started working out to overcome our biggest insecurity when we were younger, which was our self-confidence. You may be going through some challenges right now, or you may want to get fit, and we can certainly relate.

We always kind were interested in the health & fitness world and wanted to gain some muscle due to the numerous bullying in our teenage years. We figured we could do something about how our body appears. It was the beginning of our transformation journey. We had no idea where to start, but we both just got started. We felt worried and afraid at times that other people would make fun of us for doing the exercises the wrong way. We always wished we had a friend to guide us and who could show us the ropes.

After a lot of work, studying, and countless trials and errors. Some people began to notice how we were both getting more fit and how we were starting to form a keen interest in the topic. It led many friends and new faces to come to us and ask us for fitness advice. At first, it seemed odd when people asked us to help them get in shape. But what kept us going is when they started to see changes in their own body and told us it's the first time that they saw real results! From there, more people kept coming to us, and it made both of us realize after so much reading and studying in this field that it did help us, but it also allowed us to help others. To date, we have coached and trained numerous clients who have achieved some pretty amazing results.

Today, both of us own & operate this publishing business, where we bring passionate and expert authors to write about health and fitness topics. We also run an online fitness business, and we would love to connect with you by inviting you to visit the website on the following page and signing up for our e-mail newsletter (you will even get a free book).

Last but not least, if you are in the position we were once in and you want some guidance, don't hesitate and ask. I will be there to help you out!

Your coaches,

Alex &George Kaplo

Download another book for Free

We want to thank you for purchasing this book and offer you another book (just as long and valuable as this book), "Health & Fitness Mistakes You Don't Know You're Making," completely free.

Visit the link below to sign-up and receive it:

www.effingopublishing.com/gift

In this book, we will break down the most common health & fitness mistakes, you are probably committing right now, and will reveal how you can quickly get in the best shape of your life!

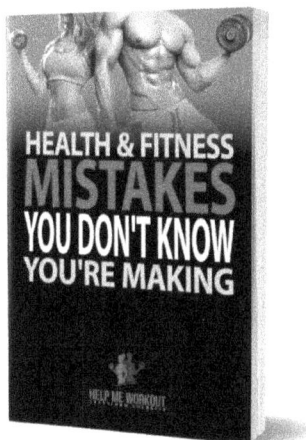

In addition to this valuable gift, you will also have an opportunity to get our new books for free, enter giveaways, and receive other useful emails from us. Again, visit the link to sign up:

www.effingopublishing.com/gift

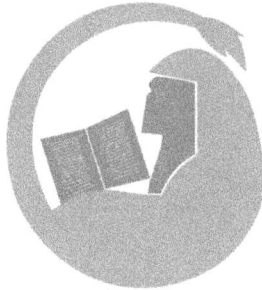

EFFINGO
Publishing

For more great books visit:

EffingoPublishing.com